You've Got This

Also by K. Susanne Jones:

The Hot Flash Relief Guide
Get Relief from the Power Surges

Magic Without Spells
The Complete Series

Before You Click 'Publish'
Self-Publishing On Amazon for Beginners

Join the Community:

Facebook: *www.facebook.com/ksjonesauthor*

Twitter: *@ajonesgirl*

Blog: *www.ajonesgirl.com*

Email: *ksjones@ajonesgirl.com*

You've Got This

Mind Hacks for Surviving Cancer Treatment

K. Susanne Jones

YOU'VE GOT THIS; MIND HACKS FOR
SURVIVING CANCER TREATMENT
Text Copyright © 2014 KS Jones
All Rights Reserved

First CreateSpace Edition

ISBN: 1503328627
ISBN-13: 978-1503328624

To my community. To say that I wouldn't have survived without you is an understatement.

CONTENTS

Forward

Most of the tips I want to share with you will be about getting through treatment mentally and emotionally, but every so often I'll share a little something that helped with my symptoms. In those cases, I urge you with all of my heart to talk to your doctors and nurses before trying anything – certain treatments have interactions with over-the-counter medications or herbal supplements. Also, everyone reacts differently to remedies, so work closely with your medical team to see what ideas might work safely for you without having an adverse effect on your treatment.

"Run when you can, walk if you have to, crawl if you must; just never give up."

Welcome to the Club

"It's not what we'd hoped..."

On May 12, 2013 – Mother's Day – I found a lump the size of a small orange just behind the nipple of my left breast. Disbelief, shock, denial and terror flooded my brain as I stared helplessly at my kids watching TV in the next room. My kids...oh my god, my kids, I thought.

I ran to my computer and searched for descriptions of what different breast lumps felt like. If I could find a description of something totally harmless and benign that fit my lump, I would feel better. I'd still get it checked, but I'd feel better. But nothing feels like cancer except cancer. So nothing on any of the sites described my lump except the final entry of every list. Cancer.

Two weeks and two biopsies later, on May 28, 2013, I was diagnosed with invasive ductal carcinoma. The tumor turned out to be 6.5cm x 7.0cm x 3.0cm, which in layman's terms means really, really huge. I chose to have a bilateral mastectomy, which then revealed six lymph nodes also affected by cancer cells. A PET scan had shown no metastases anywhere else in my body, so with all the pomp and circumstance of a footnote on

1

my pathology report, I was declared Stage IIIa. I had stage 3 cancer. It still doesn't compute.

They tend to throw the book at breast cancer in women under 40 (I was 38), and tend to *really* throw the book at stage 3 cancer in general, so after I had recovered from my mastectomy, I faced five months of chemo, then six weeks of radiation, reconstruction surgeries, and now ten years of the drug tamoxifen, which restricts my supply of estrogen and helps to prevent a recurrence. By now I know most of the lab techs by name, the surgery risk sheet by heart, and can rattle off my health record number and birthdate like a pro. I can spot newbies on the chemo floor from twenty paces – they're the ones with that dazed and wary look in their eyes, like they're waiting to wake up from a bad dream.

Those are my stats – my credentials, as it were. That's what allows me to publish a book in the "Cancer" section without a bunch of letters after my name. But you know full well that this information doesn't tell the story of what I went through. In those moments on May 28, as I sat listening to a surgeon tell me I had cancer, staring a hole through the magazine next to me and holding back the frightened tears as best I could, a new person was being formed. A new version of myself was being created.

As I sit here at my computer trying to get everything organized into a story I can tell, I still get lost in the memories. There are times when something trips me up and I find myself staring into space for a few minutes, frozen in a memory. We are forever changed, you and I. We cannot go back and forget the sound of the person's voice who told us, "You have cancer". My goal all the way through treatment was to make sure the version of me who came out the other end of the tunnel was stronger, softer, more flexible and resilient than the person who was dragged inside. I wanted to make sure the experience wasn't wasted on me.

That might sound a bit crazy.

But here's the thing, I've heard tons of stories of people who have been diagnosed with cancer, and very few of them start with the words, "I was living such a happy and fulfilling life, then out of nowhere I was diagnosed with cancer." Most stories start out with their own list of horrors the person was going through when they were diagnosed. Loss of a loved one, loss of a job, family disputes...the list goes on and on. Personally I was in the middle of an ugly divorce and bankruptcy process. I was a single mother with a job I didn't like, fighting with my ex and his mother over money and power and past injuries. When the diagnosis came through, all I could think was, "Are you kidding me?! I don't have time for this!"

You might have had a similar reaction or a completely opposite one, but either way I'm betting there were things in your life that you weren't happy or satisfied with. And I might get an eyebrow for saying this, but my theory is that sometimes we get onto the wrong path and the Universe needs to shake us up. All of the hints have gone unnoticed or ignored, and it has no choice but to swoop in, scoop us up and place us on a new path. That's what my experience was, and what I held onto each time I struggled to find a point to all the pain.

What I want to give to you, why I'm writing this book, are also the *little* ways I made it through treatment. My overall attitude was that there was a reason for all of this, big things I needed to learn, but those thoughts don't always help when the fatigue and the nausea and the fear and the depression set in. My survival depended on the little things – tricks and tips and small words of encouragement that allowed me to get through one or two hours of hell so I could come up for air, *then* focus on the big stuff again. Because it's all well and good to offer swim lessons to someone who is drowning, but you have to get them out of the water where they can breathe first.

So here's me, standing on the side, offering you my humble pool noodle in hopes that during the times your head is above water you will be able to see the new person you're becoming. The stronger, softer, more resilient and beautiful person I know will be standing on the other side of this.

You can do it.

It *is* going to suck sometimes. It *is* going to hurt sometimes. There will be days you're not sure you want to make it through. But you can, and you will make it through this treatment. Do you hear me? You will make it through this treatment. Say that out loud, I don't care where you are or who might hear you – say it right now. "I will make it through this treatment."

I will make it through this treatment.

There. That's all you have to do right now. All you have to do right this second is say those words. So take a deep breath, square your shoulders and put one foot in front of the other.

4

I'm right here with you.

15 Things I Would Tell My Pre-Chemo Self If I Could

1. You've got this.

2. Don't bother buying the lint brush.

3. Some things will be cumulative, but not everything - your mental endurance will get stronger as you go.

4. Start taking Metamucil now, and don't skip a dose. Ever.

5. That feeling like you can't get out of bed, and can't eat, and hate everything and everyone around you, lasts around five to seven days per treatment cycle. That might seem like an eternity in the moment, but the important thing is that it ends each time.

6. The prescription laxative the physician's assistant wants to give you is a bad idea. A really bad idea.

7. So is the enema.

8. It's okay to feel good when you feel good; no one is going to yell at you and say you should be back at work.

9. The hair loss is going to be harder than you

think, and you'll handle it better than you thought you would.

10. Showers will be cold though.

11. Your kids are awesome people, and will show you what big, resilient hearts they have. They will force you out of bed on some days, jump in and curl up with you on others, and forgive you for the moments when you're tired and nauseous and discouraged, and you lose your mind and scream at them so hard your throat hurts.

12. Get your hands out of your mouth.

13. Heartburn = nausea. Treat the heartburn, help the nausea.

14. That instinct you had not to delete a bunch of people from your Facebook friends list...that was a good one. So was accepting Christina's offer to go with you to treatments.

15. You've got this. I promise, you really do.

Section 1, Save Your Knees

*"Life is 10% what happens to you and 90% how
you respond to it."* ~Charles R Swindoll

Let me get one thing out there right off the
bat – I am not a doctor, nurse, or medical
professional in any capacity.

I went through just over a year and a half of
cancer treatments, which means I've learned a holy
heck of a lot of medical terms and can read a
pathology report like nobody's business, but I will
not be giving you medical advice here – that's for
your medical team to do.

What I will be giving you is advice about
how to save your knees. Let me explain…

Every so often a pregnant friend or
acquaintance will ask me for advice about morning
sickness. I had horrible morning sickness (read: all
day sickness) with both of my children, so it stands
to reason I'd have words of wisdom on how to
battle it. But I only ever have one piece of wisdom
for them.

Put a step stool next to every toilet in your
house, so that you have something to sit on.

Will this make your morning sickness go
away? No. Will it save your knees when you're
running to the toilet every half hour, sometimes

staying there for twenty minutes waiting for the wave of nausea to pass? Yes. Yes, it will. And that is all I was ever able to do for myself when I was pregnant. I tried everything out there, from sucking on ginger candy to sipping ginger ale to chewing on raw ginger in the middle of the grocery store (not recommended). I made sure to eat small meals every two hours, I stayed away from spicy foods, and I kept moving. Those things made it bearable (and helped during chemo too, by the way), but they did not make it go away. The most valuable lesson I ever learned during the morning sickness months was to save my knees.

That's what I want to give you here.

There are a ton of good books and websites out there with medical advice on how to handle symptoms and recovery periods. Your doctors and nurses and pharmacists will have good advice too. What this book is for are the mental and emotional challenges you have ahead of you, and the small things you can do to get your head above water on a bad day. You may breeze through chemo with nary a whiff of nausea or fatigue (I kinda hate you if you do), or walk away from a bilateral mastectomy taking nothing but a couple of ibuprofen (please don't even tell me if that's what you did), but you are still living through cancer treatment, and that comes with a level of gravity that treatment for other conditions doesn't always have.

You may or may not end up *looking* like you have cancer (not everyone loses their hair during chemo, for example, and not all cancer treatments even include chemotherapy), but the word "cancer" has been said in the same sentence as the word "you". That does a number on your mind and emotions. It changes you for the rest of your life. Everything will now be measured in terms of before and after that moment when someone told you that you have cancer.

My life is forever altered, and I wouldn't change it for anything in the world. I have survived, and my life is richer for it.

Let's begin.

Sources of Strength

"Survivors are like tea bags; you don't know how strong we are until you put us in hot water."

Okay, so you've survived your diagnosis. Well done. Seriously, well done. You are now officially a survivor. From here on out, regardless of your treatment plan, regardless of how your body reacts to that treatment, you are a survivor. You have survived hearing words that can break the will of the strongest person out there, so in my eyes you are a hero and an inspiration.

Get used to hearing that.

I'm going to start by helping you find your Source of Strength – SOS for short. Your SOS is an image or phrase or memory or affirmation that can lift you out of hell no matter what. It's going to be the life ring you grab when you feel overwhelmed and scared. It's going to be the reminder to square your shoulders and get back up again. It's going to be what forces you to open that door and walk through it, even though every muscle in your body wants to run away. Because you're going to have to learn to do that. You're going to get really good at it actually.

Mine was my kids. Not just the thought of them, but the thought, "What would I be feeling right now if it was one of them who was battling cancer?" My answer was immediate and loud – I'd wish it were me. I'd be *begging* the Universe to give it to me, let me go through it instead of them. 'I'll take it, I'll take all of it, thank you for giving it to me instead of them.' That thought would give me literally a punch of strength.

So I would have my pity party – I would cry a little, deny a lot, rage a bit…and then that thought would force its way into my mind and I'd be back in the game.

Quotes

Another SOS for me was a list of quotes about strength and courage. The morning of my mastectomy I was literally shaking with fear, I had to talk myself through the entire process of getting dressed and into the car like you'd talk to a frightened child. "It's okay, just focus on getting dressed, you'll be okay…" and the like. I sobbed as I tried to write a letter to my ex-husband about how I wanted things handled with our kids if I didn't make it through the surgery. My mind cycled over and over on how I was going to feel afterward and whether I had done everything I could to prepare for the recovery, and how I was going to cover up my swollen eyes and the choking "sup-sups" my diaphragm was making from crying so hard. Then I caught sight of a quote I had scribbled down earlier.

"Sometimes having courage just means showing up."

I let out a breath and felt my shoulders drop about three inches. That's all I had to do, just show up. All I had to do was walk out the door and get into the car – I didn't even have to drive since my mother was giving me a ride to the hospital. That's all. It was okay to be terrified – *it didn't mean I wasn't strong*. And unlike an interview or audition or even the first day of a new job, there wasn't really anything I had to do once I got there – the nurses, surgeons, and anesthesiologists would be the ones doing the work.

I looked at that quote before every single chemo treatment. All I had to do was walk through the door of the treatment room – the rest was up to the nurses and pharmacists. Sometimes when everything is a bit overwhelming, it's a relief to hand it over. All of the strength you have can be used to put your hand out and push open the door, then to move your legs forward until you reach the chair.

My fourth chemo cycle was like that – I walked through the door and sat down, then closed my eyes and let it all go. The nurse did the rest. It was a bit out of character for me to do that, since I was usually very chatty and positive. But that day was hard – I knew what was coming, and I knew that no matter what I did I was going to feel like complete hell by the time we were in the car on the way home. So I let myself off the hook and put what little strength I had toward staying in that chair.

I've included my favorite quotes about strength and courage throughout this book. Feel free to snatch them up for your own. Pull them out when you feel lost and overwhelmed, or scared and angry.

You may already have a couple of ideas for your own SOS's, or you may be thinking, "For the love of Pete, how do I figure that out?!" Hang on, I'll give you some suggestions.

Ask

First, I want you to *ask* for your SOS. Ask God, the Universe, or just ask your own brain for something to give you strength. Ask. Allow your mind to start working on the problem without inhibiting it with doubts. Just take a deep breath, close your eyes, and ask.

"What can I use as a source of strength in my most challenging moments?"

Now what was the first thing that popped into your head? Was it something that made you laugh? Was it something that made you cry? Was it something so random you're left with the thought, "Well, that didn't work…"

It did work. It's still working.

Your mind is on the job, putting together ideas for what you can use. The Universe is on the job, organizing future events to place you in front of what you need. Pay attention over the next day or week to what shows up. And continue to ask for more.

Past Experience

Another way of finding SOS's is to take a moment and remember a really challenging time you've already lived through. Think back to the hardest part of that time period or event. In hindsight, what helped you cope? You survived it, since you're here now reading this, so something got you through. What was it? Is it something you can also use now?

Mantras

Look for positive affirmations you can repeat to yourself as mantras. If you find your brain on overdrive – especially at night when you're trying to get some much-needed sleep – repeat the mantra either out loud or in your mind to break the cycle of negative or scary thoughts. Some of my favorites are below.

"I can do this."

"With every breath, my muscles relax and my mind clears."

"My mind is clear and my body is healed."

"My body is healing, every second of every day."

"I am healthy. I am healed."

Gratitude

The quickest way I've found to shift out of a negative thought pattern is through gratitude. And the quickest way to turn gratitude into an SOS is to take the statement of what you need and throw the words "Thank you" in front of it. "I need the strength to go to my first chemo treatment" becomes, "Thank you for the strength I need to make myself go to my first chemo treatment." "I need patience to keep from punching this idiot in the mouth" becomes, "Thank you for the patience I need to keep from punching this idiot in the mouth." And so on.

You may find several SOS's or use only one, or you may find that each type of treatment you face requires a completely different kind of SOS. Keep yourself open to new SOS's as you go along – there's nothing wrong with keeping that particular cupboard stocked.

Your Happy Place

"Courage doesn't always roar. Sometimes courage is the little voice at the end of the day that says, 'I'll try again tomorrow.'"

I've read in more places than I can count how valuable yoga and meditation can be during cancer treatments, particularly chemotherapy. I was able to find a way to meditate eventually, and it was of great value because it helped me slow down and live one day at a time. It helped me get into the driver's seat of my life and stop being a victim.

But I'm going to be honest with you, it didn't really happen until after the worst of my chemo treatments had passed.

I had five months of chemotherapy – four cycles of A/C (Adriamyocin & Cytoxine) every other week, then twelve weekly cycles of taxol. During the A/C cycles, the first week I was a mess, the second week I was fine. Then rinse, repeat for eight weeks. During the taxol cycles, I was a mess for a day or two, mostly from the steroid they gave me, then fine except for fatigue the rest of the week.

Now, by the end of twelve weeks of taxol the fatigue was bad enough that "fine except for fatigue" meant "walking through molasses twenty-four hours a day", but there was no nausea, bone pain, reflux or constipation to worry about. It was during the taxol cycles that I was able to learn how to meditate and when I did the majority of my mental healing.

Before then, I was the person drowning who needed a life preserver, not swim lessons.

During the A/C cycles I used a couple of techniques I had learned while preparing for the birth of my first child (I studied Hypnobirthing). One of them is incredibly simple – just find your happy place.

Sounds a little too easy, right? Actually it can be as simple or as complicated as you choose. It takes preparation though, and a little practice. If you aren't in the habit of visualization, or if you've never really thought about visualization before, give it a shot right now.

I want you to look at your thumb. Just look at it for a minute, noting the nail, your skin, any scars or hangnails you might have. Then close your eyes, take a deep breath, and picture your thumb.

There. Did you picture it? You've just practiced visualization.

If you were able to picture even the shape of your thumb, you were successful. If you were able to picture every line in your knuckle, then holy cow, way to go. Whatever level of detail your mind pulled up, this is how you will get a break from the hard moments. You're going to find a soothing image or memory to pull up and visualize when you feel your mind going into overdrive. When you start having thoughts like, "I can't do this," or "It's never going to end," you will be able to give yourself a short reprieve, and hopefully a bit of a reset button by visualizing your happy place.

During a time when you're feeling good (or at least not horrible), think of a moment in your past when you were totally relaxed and happy. Maybe it's from your childhood, maybe it's from a vacation you took just before you were diagnosed, but find that moment. Looking at your baby for the first time, swinging so high you felt like you were flying, cuddling with your partner when you were first falling in love, lying in the grass looking at the clouds on a warm spring day.

For me it was floating in the ocean in Florida. The sand is white there, and the water is warm and a vivid blue-green. It stays incredibly shallow for twenty-five to thirty feet, so you can walk way out and sit down and your head and shoulders are still above water. I would float on my back watching the sky, letting the gentle waves push me slowly back to the beach.

To make visualization easier, keep your images mobile – move through your visualization instead of trying to focus on a stationary object or location. Also try and recall as many details as you can. Is it warm or cold? What sounds can you hear? What colors can you see? Really feel yourself in that moment, lock it in so you can pull it up easily. I'll go so far as to suggest you start each day with that image, so that recalling it is as easy as breathing.

Then, if you find yourself cycling into negative thoughts and panic, close your eyes and go to your happy place. Stay there as long as you are able, let it sooth you and put you back into a state of calm. Then open your eyes, pull yourself up, and get back in the game.

What You Need

"Put your own oxygen mask on first… then *assist others."*

Regardless of where you are in your diagnosis or treatment, you have to put yourself first. If you don't put your oxygen mask on before you try and help someone else, you will pass out and be useless to everyone.

My biggest challenge was learning to be honest. It's not like I was a big liar before I got cancer, but I wasn't particularly good at recognizing what I needed and then demanding that either. I was the queen of the white lie – "No no, I'm fine, you do what you need to do and I'll work around it…"

I was also very good at accepting awful circumstances and braving my way through them. Or justifying why having things be hard was somehow good for me. In my divorce, my job, my relationships with my friends and family, I prided myself in my ability to roll with it when horrible things happened.

Then one day I was driving and there was a pothole in front of me. I braced for impact and heard the familiar mantra start in my brain, where I hoped my tire would be okay but understood that there was probably a higher reason if not. But this time I noticed something – the car in front of me swerved to miss the pothole. And suddenly this pothole and my victim mentality around it became a symbol of everything that was wrong in my way of thinking. Why the hell wasn't I swerving to miss the bad stuff?

That stupid pothole became a catalyst for changing my entire approach to life.

It's okay to say no. It's okay to want your sister at your appointments instead of your husband. It's okay to tell your over-reactive friend to go find someone else to vent to. It's okay. This cancer thing? You're going to have to roll with that, but what you put up with and who you surround yourself with are completely in your control.

A survivor friend told me about her chemo experience – in her infusion room people were grouped together so they saw each other at every treatment, and her group became pretty close. She said that folks pretty much fell into two categories – the jokesters and the sour pusses. The jokesters would laugh about what they were going through, leave funny messages for each other on the ceiling, and talk about how beautiful their fake boobs would be when they were ninety. The sour pusses considered that behavior to be completely inappropriate and resented the jokes and the laughter. Ten years later they attempted to have a reunion, and sought out everyone who had been in their little group. Most of the jokesters were still around and cancer free, but not one of the sour pusses had made it.

Do what you will with *that* information.

Your reactions to things are in your control. You can love one idea about an upcoming treatment (time off of work, whoo hoo!) and hate another. Or love and hate something simultaneously – I mourn the loss of my breasts every day, but love that I don't have to wear a bra anymore.

Before I started chemo, everyone (including me) expected me to go get a cute pixie haircut in preparation for being bald. My hair at that time was really long, so we all thought it would ease the transition and give me control over something at a time when I didn't have control over much. I tried. I started to call several places to make an appointment, but would hang up before anyone answered. As time went on I created excuses – I couldn't find a place I trusted, it was too expensive, I was going to Vegas for my sister's bachelorette weekend so I wanted to keep it for that trip, etc. But the truth was, I just couldn't do it. I realized that I *wanted* to keep my hair as long as possible, and that I was okay shaving it all off at once when it started to fall out. Making that decision was a huge relief. It was such a minor thing but it felt good to allow myself to have that opinion – I didn't want to cut my hair. Deciding *not* to cut my hair was more empowering to me than cutting it.

Do what *you* need, not what is expected of you or what society thinks is supposed to happen. Make cancer jokes if that's your style, flirt with the phlebotomist who does your blood draw every week, pick out a crazy pink wig instead of a normal one. Or do none of those things, even though society or your friends and family think you should.

Whatever you need to do to make this experience a little less horrifying, do that.

Denial...Not Just a River in Egypt

Denial gets a bad rap sometimes. Yes, it's a bad thing if you get a cancer diagnosis and pretend it didn't happen and don't get treatment (note – deciding not to get cancer treatment after careful research and soul searching is a totally different thing). But denial exists to give our brains and our hearts a break.

You know those first few moments in the morning, when you're not quite awake yet, but not asleep anymore either? In those moments you don't remember that you have cancer. Your heart feels light and easy and the day is bright and full of possibilities. I cherish those moments. Then the memories rush in, the day's tasks loom in front of you...but underneath it all your heart got a break, and that can't be a bad thing.

The first week after my diagnosis I had another level of denial; I developed an irrational...I guess hope, or fear, that I'd get a call from the surgeon telling me the second biopsy came back negative – the first biopsy had been misdiagnosed and I didn't actually have cancer. And how embarrassing it would be to have to tell everyone it was all a mistake. Obviously I would celebrate like crazy, but this weird part of me would be really embarrassed for putting everyone through all that fear when it wasn't real. And that same little weird part of me couldn't stop thinking about it. Which grief animal is that, I thought. Denial? Bargaining? Do they have a step called Delusional?

Looking back, that was my brain putting a buffer between my diagnosis and me. I avoided long brooding sessions thinking about who would raise my kids by brooding on how embarrassing it would be to tell people it had been a mistake.

There were days when it was all just too much – the gravity of the word 'cancer', the emotions of everyone around me, the things I was supposed to be doing that were just unreal…it was too much. I'd find myself saying, "I can't…I just…can't right now." On those days it was healthier to take a break and watch dumb TV, or go for a walk, or just go grocery shopping – the more mundane and routine the better. Even now, when things get overwhelming, sometimes I literally just vacuum the house or organize a file cabinet. Something that can take enough of my attention to give my mind and my heart a break, but doesn't require a huge amount of brain power.

Preparing for my last surgery, the reconstruction that gave me soft and squishy boobs instead of rock-hard tissue expanders, was in some ways just as traumatic as my double mastectomy. Partly because of a residual shell-shock I feel about surgery in general now, and partly because I knew what was coming and was dreading the recovery period. I had to tackle those preparations in small chunks. On one day I pulled out the front-clasp sports bras and mastectomy corsets to have them ready, but even seeing them again sent me reeling. So I stopped there. I put them in an easy-to-access drawer and walked away. The next day I brought the recliner into my bedroom in anticipation of not being able to sleep on my side for a long time, but again, I had to stop there and walk away. I got everything ready that I needed to, but one small task at a time, sometimes only one task per day.

It's okay to feel like you need a break. And it's okay to *take* that break. Don't skip doctor's appointments or anything, but take a break when you need it. And it's okay when denial shows up. It's healthy in light doses, and it's a part of all of this – you're not crazy. Allow it – take a good look at it, determine if it's something that can help or hurt you, then let it do its job.

The Word 'Should'

"Of all the saddest words of tongue or pen, the saddest are these, "It might have been." ~John Greenleaf Whittier

This one isn't particularly easy, and is something I have to remind myself to work on every day. But if you can master it, or even just improve a little, you'll save yourself mountains of grief.

You've got to get the words 'should' and 'shouldn't' out of your vocabulary. 'I *shouldn't* have cancer', 'It *shouldn't* be this hard', 'I *should* be feeling better by now', 'I *should* be able to work all the way through treatment', 'S/he *should* be more supportive'. The list goes on and on, and will torture you if you let it.

There is no such thing as what 'should' be, only what *is* and what *can be*.

I believe with every ounce of my soul that life is what you create as you go. I believe wholeheartedly in what *can* be. To do that though, I have to get rid of any sense of what *should* be. 'Should' is a judgmental word full of criticism and negativity and doubt. Even when used in the future tense, "I should be able to finish that by noon", it's got a negative tone to it.

You've got to focus on what *is*. Are you feeling like crap right now? Are you in pain? That's what *is*. And once you recognize and get a good look at what *is* then you can start to try and change it into what *can* be.

If you stay on the thought of what 'should be', you'll never get to a place where you can move forward. But if you eliminate 'should' and 'shouldn't', anything is possible.

"I shouldn't have cancer" becomes "I have cancer, but I can beat it."

"It shouldn't be this hard" becomes "This is hard, and I'm strong enough to get through it."

"I should be feeling better by now" becomes "I'm still in pain, what can I do to fix it?"

"I should be able to work all the way through treatment' becomes "I'm going to *try* to keep working through treatment."

"S/he should be more supportive" becomes "S/he's not as supportive as I need her/him to be, can I ask someone else for help?"

The word 'should' keeps you in the hole; recognizing what is and what can be gives you a ladder to get out.

Tears

"Let your tears come. Let them water your soul."
~Eileen Mayhew

I cry in the car a lot. It seems to be the only time my brain will give up control and let my heart have the reigns. It's also the time I get to listen to music without interruption. I've trained my kids that on trips longer than a few minutes, mommy needs "quiet time", and we all daydream and listen to music as we get from one place to another.

In the weeks after my diagnosis, my commute to and from work was a regular therapy session. I'd drop the kids off at school and daycare and then just let the tears flow – I would have to reapply my makeup in the parking lot before going inside. I'd also feel a little better and more able to tackle the day.

My dad passed away in 1997, and my mom talks about how she'd let herself cry for a while, then after a bit she'd tell herself, "That's enough," and get up and do something else. That's basically what my commute therapy was, because it had to end when I arrived at my destination. I let myself cry as hard as I needed to, then squared my shoulders and got out of the car.

I also had to learn to let myself cry in front of other people. That was a hard one for me. I've always said I'll tell a stranger on a park bench my entire life story, but even my closest friends never hear how I feel about any of it. I began by opening up to random nurses and lab techs who I'd never see again, many of whom would open up to me with their own survival stories. Eventually I talked to friends and family, and when I felt my voice cracking and the tears welling up, I didn't stop. Some folks were more comfortable than others with this, and not everyone responded with exactly the right words, but for me it was about *my* learning curve, and learning to cry when I felt like crying.

Something nice that has happened with this new crying-in-front-of-people thing is that I feel stronger. When I'm able to let down my guard and allow the tears to come, it's like a big middle finger to the critical voice inside who thinks showing emotion makes you weak. My dad told me once the thing he liked best about me was that I was quick to smile. Well, now I'm quick to cry too – and I love that about myself.

Forgiving You

"It just wouldn't be a picnic without the ants."

Here's the thing; you have cancer, and that sucks. I can't even describe to you how much that sucks. It's unfair, and you shouldn't have to be going through this. And guess what, it's okay to feel that way. It's okay to have days when it feels truly unfair, because it is. Should you try and keep a positive attitude most of the time? Yes, overall your attitude will determine how well and how long you survive this, but you have to give yourself a break once in a while and admit that this whole cancer thing is a load of crap.

Cancer sucks on a cataclysmic level and there's no way our brains can process that level of suckage all at once. Sometimes I find myself focusing on small annoying things with a ferocity I don't understand, until I realize it's all in there, all of the suckage, and my mind is pulling out little things one at a time and allowing me to process it in chunks.

Let's face it, if you're in the middle of any traumatic event just getting out of bed in the morning can take herculean effort. Paralyzed by fear, or fatigue, or pain, or nausea...there were mornings I would lie there and wonder, what's the point? The world won't end if I just roll over and go back to sleep. Of course that would mean the kids stay home with me today because they'd miss school…sigh…okay, I'm up, I'm up…

If you're reading this, then that means you woke up this morning, *and* picked up this book, *and* started reading. Let me be the first to congratulate you - well done. If that's the only thing you accomplish today…then well done. I salute you.

Do what you can do each day and let that be enough.

Forgive yourself for being afraid…

"If you're going through hell, keep going."
~Winston Churchill

The first time I walked into the oncology building I was terrified. I felt like a stray dog being walked to the euthanasia room – I put one foot in front of the other because I had to, but every muscle in my body wanted to turn around and run back to the car. In the waiting room I scanned every other person for signs of chemo side effects. I looked everywhere for someone without hair – I wanted to see it but I didn't want to see it but I wanted to see it.

We are all going to have different reactions to each piece of this journey, and whatever you're feeling is totally okay.

A fellow survivor on my cancer forum told us about her first trip to chemotherapy – she literally ran out of the room and had to be walked back in by her daughter. This stuff is scary, it's so much scarier than probably anything you've ever had to face before. Or maybe you have faced it before, which makes it even scarier.

I talked earlier about how frightened I was before my mastectomy, but before my reconstruction surgery – over a year later – I was just as terrified. At my pre-op appointment, I walked in feeling perfectly confident, then spotted packages of pre-surgery cleansing wipes sitting on the counter for me to take home. They're not a very big deal, just big sterile cloths that you wipe your body down with the night before and the morning of any major surgery. But seeing them brought back such a giant flashback of my mastectomy experience that when the nurse came back in with the blood pressure cart, she found me curled up in the chair holding my knees to my chest and trying to slow down my breathing.

What you're going through is downright horrifying sometimes. Many things will get easier as you go – your second trip to chemo is much easier than the first, and so on. Some things won't, I'm not going to lie to you. But being strong doesn't mean not being afraid. Being strong means being terrified, but doing what needs to be done anyway.

...for hating some parts of the journey...

My last treatment cycle of A/C – the chemo cocktail that made me so sick – I was bitter and angry. It was my last one, so everyone wanted to celebrate that I was done with my first round of chemo. I had no interest in celebrating – I still had a week and a half of hell to live through. And I was just…pissed. A friend of mine made a great observation, she pointed out that since it was my last one I could allow myself to hate it – I didn't have to rally at the end of it and gear up for another one, I could just hate it. So I did. And at my next treatment when I started taxol (which didn't make me as sick), that's when I celebrated.

Radiation was another thing I hated. It was the last portion of my treatment, and came almost a year after my diagnosis, so I was beyond procedure-weary. I nearly decided to skip it, I was so sick of treatments. Plus, it involved driving forty minutes each way every day (minus weekends) for six weeks. It didn't help that my plastic surgeon was worried about whether my skin would be able to handle reconstruction after having radiation. I hated driving all that way for a five-minute procedure. I hated the six different kinds of lotion I had to use to try and keep my skin healthy, while they purposefully exposed me to something I would avoid at all costs if I didn't have stupid cancer.

The other thing I got really angry about was how much my kids had to give up. My daughter's fourth birthday fell in the middle of my chemo treatments, and we nearly had to forgo having a birthday party for her in fear of exposing me to too many germs. We couldn't have playdates at our house because I couldn't control what other kids touched and sneezed on. I dragged myself out of the house for my son's basketball games, but I couldn't take him out for ice cream afterwards because I needed to get back to bed.

It's okay to hate what you're going through. This whole process is very similar to the grieving process, and anger is definitely a part of that. You're probably angry that you have cancer, yes, but you also might be angry that you have to lose your hair, or angry that the damned hot flashes are happening every hour on the hour. It's okay. Just don't let yourself get dragged down by it – let yourself feel it and then take a deep breath and move on.

…for feeling like crap…

"I know God will not give me anything I can't handle. I just wish that He didn't trust me so much." ~Mother Teresa

I had to forgive myself for not being able to do much with my kids. For several months all I could do is make sure they were fed, got enough sleep, and took showers often enough so that they didn't smell. I had help from my family and friends – the kids and I had moved in with my mother before my mastectomy, and she's an awesome grandma. Plus, I had a few friends who would come get them for outings every so often. Somehow I dragged myself to basketball practice and games twice a week.

We also watched a lot of TV and movies together, and had popcorn and hot chocolate for dinner sometimes, and cuddled in my bed together on days I couldn't quite make it up. At the time I felt guilty, but just had to forgive myself and remember that it wasn't going to last forever.

You're probably not going to be able to be the president of your PTA during treatment, or take on that important project at work (if you're able to work through treatment). All of that will have to wait while you get healthy.

...for not being able to think clearly...

Even before your treatments begin you'll have to give yourself a break, because your brain isn't going to function normally.

In between my diagnosis and my mastectomy, I was a mess. I was tired all the time, I couldn't focus, I was losing things and forgetting simple pieces of information. I was a wreck, but I wasn't sick. Yeah I had cancer, but I wasn't *sick* – other than the weird twinges and pains in my boob from the tumor bumping into a few nerves, I had no outward symptoms. So why couldn't I function?

Because the word cancer is like a stoplight in your brain – everything comes to a raging halt as soon as the word is uttered. Then as you try to move forward, the knowledge that you have cancer and everything that comes with that remains in your field of vision, and it's hard to see around it. Like a giant billboard in the middle of the road that flashes CANCER in neon. Eventually you can adjust, and with enough time you learn to shove the flashing billboard off to the side a bit. But especially in the beginning, you're just going to be a bit scattered.

So I made lots of lists, and wrote everything down. If someone at work asked me to do something for them but I wasn't at my desk, I asked them to email me their request because I was going to forget by the time I made it to...where was I going again?

And I forgave myself. I accepted as best I could that it was going to be a while before I was back to being 100%.

...for *not* feeling like crap...

Something else you might deal with are the days you feel good. In between chemo cycles, or in between different treatment methods, you might feel completely back to yourself. And that can be weird. If you're away from work on disability, it might even bring out a bit of guilt.

It's okay to feel good on days you feel good. It's also okay to feel good but not jump right back into your routine if you don't want to. I struggled with this – I was on disability from work and had a million people chipping in to help me with my kids. So when I hit a zone where I felt fine, I didn't know what to do with myself. I wanted to scour my house and take my kids to the zoo, but didn't want my coworkers to hear about it and be frustrated that I wasn't at work. Or sometimes I felt good but really just wanted to hang out and watch TV anyway, and felt guilty that I wasn't scouring my house and taking the kids to the zoo. In the end, no one judged me for doing what I needed to do – they were happy when I felt good, and supportive when I felt like crap.

Do what you need to do in each moment and try not to worry about what other people will think. But above all, forgive yourself.

Gratitude

"Praise the bridge that carried you over."
~George Colman

When I get really frustrated and feel like everyone and everything is out to get me, I try to stop, take a breath, and say my thank you's. I find one thing I can be grateful for, and really focus on that. Sometimes what I feel grateful for is that this obstacle in front of me is going to make me stronger, or that I still have my children with me, or that I had the strength not to choke the life out of that idiot at the gas station. Whatever works, just find that one thing.

Very often once I've found one thing I'm grateful for, more things will pop into my head. Suddenly I'll remember how much it meant to me when a friend cooked several meals and filled my freezer with them. Or I'll remember how much my mother does for me every day. At the very least I can usually get myself off of the negativity train and onto a more positive outlook. At the most I can end up a blubbering mess as I realize all of the beautiful things and people I have around me.

Sometimes it just takes one little thought of gratitude to jostle you out of a negative thinking pattern.

I also practice meditation and manifestation, so in particularly frustrating times I purposefully feel grateful for something that isn't necessarily in my hands yet. As I type this one of the incisions from my most recent surgery is having a little trouble healing up, because that's the side that went through radiation and my skin just isn't the same on that side. So when I'm feeling scared or frustrated about that I say to myself, "Thank you for my healing." I imagine a beautiful white light radiating out from inside my breast, and feel grateful for my perfect skin and for my body's ability to heal completely.

I have also been known to take a breath and think, "Thank you for the patience I need to survive my children's bickering" or, "Thank you for the money I need to pay for this stupid parking ticket." It works for all kinds of things.

Have you ever heard the phrase, "It can always get worse"? To find that thing you're grateful for, maybe you need to think of how your situation could be worse. Don't spend too much time there or you'll end up walking down that road, but just for a second think of someone worse off than you, and take a moment to be grateful you aren't that person. Maybe it's someone whose cancer is much worse than yours, or someone with more financial hardships. Or maybe it's someone who's loved ones you can't imagine having to deal with. Allow yourself to be grateful for your own life, grateful for *your* hardships, because you couldn't possibly deal with theirs.

When you can shift yourself to a feeling of gratitude, it will pull you out of the muck. We all have one thing we can be grateful for in each moment, and once you find that one thing most of the time more will pop up and make themselves noticed. Then you can wrap those around you and keep marching.

Prognosis

"Once you choose hope, anything's possible."
~Christopher Reeve

I very purposefully never asked for my prognosis. In my case, there wasn't really a formal prognosis anyhow, because everything in the cancer world my doctors live in seems to work off of five-year survival rates. Treatments were recommended based on their ability to decrease my chances of having a recurrence in the next five years. Once I reach five years' post-treatment, they'll just be looking at the next five years. I imagine it's a little different for anyone who is stage IV – those with metastases in multiple locations in the body – but I don't know for certain. Other medical teams may have a different way of handling it too.

Either way, I didn't want to hear about my five-year recurrence percentages. I got annoyed when doctors would talk about five-year survival rates, even when they were telling me how great those rates were, because when I thought about survival rates I was thinking in terms of fifty years, not five.

My physical survival was non-negotiable.

So I purposefully talked about what I would do when my treatment year was over – *I made plans*. I didn't allow anyone to discuss fears about my survival in front of me. I went as far as to tell them not to even put that thought out into the Universe.

The next year was going to suck, but then it would be behind me.

I haven't lived through a grim prognosis, so I won't pretend to know what you're going through if you have. My humble suggestion though is to put it out there that your survival rate is 100%. After all, at this point – at this very moment – that's what your track record is. If you're reading this book you have survived until now. That's all any of us have, really...right? So why not let yourself be like everyone else in this aspect? Why not?

All of us should have a will and arrangements for our loved ones if we pass away suddenly. All of us should live as though there's not much time left – we should tell people we love them, do the things we dream of, hold our children tight.

Doing those things won't guarantee you'll live to see tomorrow. Doing those things doesn't mean you're giving up, either.

My father was given a six-month prognosis and put onto hospice when he was fifty-two years old. He put the deadline onto his calendar, and who knows how often he looked at it. His death came within days of that date, even though the date he had written on his calendar was actually off by a month.

A survivor I met along the way was also given a six-month prognosis, but she ignored it. She put her financial and legal affairs in order and then refused to think about it again. She greeted every day with gratitude, and smiled and laughed and joked around as often as possible. She thought of her body as healthy and healed, she visualized the doctors shaking their heads in disbelief as they pronounced her cancer free. That was three years ago, and she's been in remission for most of that time.

No matter what, do what you need to do to take care of your loved ones, but don't fixate on what your survival rate is. Focus on the future, on loving everyone as hard as you can, and on healing your body and soul.

Section II, It Takes a Village

"When everything goes to hell, the people who stand by you without flinching – they are your family. " ~Jim Butcher

In 2013 I was a single mother used to relying on myself for everything. Not because I didn't have fabulous people in my life to lean on, but because somewhere along the way I had decided I didn't need to lean on anyone. Somewhere along the way I decided I was a superhero; able to hold down a full time job, raise my two young children by myself, take care of the bills and the meals and the cleaning, all while keeping everyone around me happy.

The Universe decided to show me just how wrong I was.

My biggest lesson, my biggest learning curve, was leaning on people. Truly leaning on them. Not just for normal things like babysitting or venting sessions, but for strength to get through experiences I never even imagined I'd be facing. I had to learn how to be honest about what I needed, how to open up to people about things that scared me, and how to cry in front of the people I care about. Or perfect strangers sometimes, whoever happened to be nearby.

I had to learn that there are just some things you can't survive on your own.

No ifs ands or buts about it. You will need people around you if you want to get through this. Argue with me all you like, it's true. If you don't have a community right now, go get one. If the community you currently have is filled with assholes, go get a new one. Join a support group, book club, online cancer forum, online gaming forum I don't care, but gather people around you.

Other advice books may tell you to keep everything close to your chest; they'll tell you that you don't need constant phone calls or stories about people they knew who died of cancer, etc etc…and yes, that can be true. People can be very stupid when they get hit with big information. But I disagree that you should hide away and face this alone or face it with only one other person. In my experience the presence of a community makes or breaks your survival – both physical survival and emotional survival. Your community can help you not just survive this, but thrive afterward.

Here's the hard part though – you will have to teach your community how to take care of you.

Well-meaning people will tell you (or maybe you're thinking this yourself) that you shouldn't have to be worrying about other peoples' feelings. This is about you and your journey and *your* feelings. To that I say yes, that's absolutely true. I've been telling you throughout this book to focus on what you need. To that end, what you need right now is your community.

It takes a village to survive cancer.

Most people aren't going to know what to say, and there may be some awkward silences. Ignorant, unintentionally hurtful things are going to come out of some folks' mouths sometimes. But they are also going to be the ones who give you that tiny gem of advice that gets you through a tough day, and that will make it all worth it.

I'll give you an example.

Before I told my Facebook crowd about my diagnosis, I went through my 'friends' list and tried to weed out people who I wasn't close to. After all, I was about to go through something incredibly personal, and all of the advice books said to be selective in who I told about my diagnosis. My friends list only includes people I've met in person at some point or another, but certainly there are people on there who I haven't seen in years, or people I barely know but accepted the friend request anyhow. So I walked through each person one by one, looking at their picture and deciding how close I was to them. The funny thing is, I couldn't bring myself to unfriend even one person. Something inside just told me to hold off and wait.

One person who would have been on the delete list is a man named Dwayne. I had met him a grand total of twice, and while the one time we hung out we had talked and laughed like old friends, we hadn't really talked since. But I kept him in my community with everyone else.

One day a month or so into chemo I was having a particularly hard day. Not really any different than any other hard day, but I wasn't coping very well emotionally. So I posted on Facebook about it – generally I only posted positive things on Facebook because I wanted that crowd to be my cheerleaders, I wanted them to see me as strong and resilient so I could see myself as strong and resilient. But that day sucked, and I needed help.

"Need positive thoughts this morning, like literally, need to have positive thoughts. Feeling like crap again today and unable to keep myself from being pissed off about it. I know that in a few days I'll be fine again, but right now sucks. I guess I need to remember what another wise survivor said once – 'Who of your friends would you give this to?' No one, I'll take it. It just sucks."

I got thirty-eight comments from this post, all filled with love and laughter and people wrapping their virtual arms around me and lifting me up out of the mud. I laugh and cry every time I read them – and I still read them sometimes when I need a pick-me-up. But one comment sliced through everything and wrapped around my heart like a blanket. It was from Dwayne.

"So, we only know each other very casually, but I want you to know that I hear you. I know from your posts that you are a person of substantial fortitude. In short, you are an impressive individual...a fighter, and a winner. With that said, you have the universe's permission to go low when necessary. So do that. And it will not beat you. You'll be back. Let it blow by you, and get up and fight again when it does. Your friends, close or distant, are all rooting for you, and have your back. All peace to you, sister."

I still turn into a blubbering mess when I read that.

What he said was that it's okay to have a bad day. It doesn't mean you aren't a fighter; it doesn't mean you've been beaten. It's just a bad day, and it will pass. Those words are etched into my heart now – I carry them around like my son carries his favorite stuffed animal. I have even had the great honor of passing those words on to other friends going through tough recoveries. I'm passing them on to you now.

If I had deleted Dwayne from my friends list, I wouldn't have those words.

In this section I will teach you how to gather your community. I will teach you how to tell them what you need. How to be open and honest in each instant. And yes, how to forgive them for their clumsy and stupid moments.

Because your community has the power to lift you up and carry you through dark times if you let them.

But only if you let them.

Gather your community, tell them what you need, be as honest as possible and forgive them if necessary. You cannot make it through treatment without them.

Spreading the News

"Hope begins in the dark, the stubborn hope that if you just show up and try to do the right thing, the dawn will come." ~Anne Lamott

When it was time to tell the people in my life that I had been diagnosed with breast cancer, I struggled with how to do it. I had been talking to two of my best friends and my mother about the mammogram/ultrasound/biopsy experience, so when the surgeon called and dropped the c-word all I had to tell them was, "It wasn't what we'd hoped," and they knew the rest. Not that those were easy conversations, mind you, but they were quick and didn't require any forethought.

Everyone else however…holy crap. I know a lot of people, and they all care about me and my kids in different capacities. And none of them knew I had been going through the diagnosis process. I decided to tackle it the way I used to advise couples to do when I was a wedding coordinator – I divided everyone I knew into tiers of friendship and handled each tier separately.

My tiers were:

1) People I told immediately, either in person or on the phone.

2) People I told a few days later, mostly on the phone.

3) People I could send a group email to.

4) My Facebook crowd.

The first day...well you know what that first day is like. You can't think past the shock but somehow you get through certain tasks. My mom drove down and we went to see the surgeon together to get the preliminary game plan. Then we took the kids out to dinner so neither of us had to cook. I left the table and walked outside of the restaurant to call my sisters without my kids hearing me. Because my kids weren't even on the tier chart I had created...I still had no idea how to broach the subject with them.

I sat on the curb for a long time trying to figure out what to say. I needed to give my sisters the information in a way I could get the facts out without dissolving into a stupid sobbing mess, but in a way that wasn't cold or unfeeling either. After all, I was telling them their sister had cancer - they were going to remember this conversation the same way I remembered the surgeon's phone call to me. So I planned out a couple of sentences and then dialed.

I think I called my younger sister first (the day is still a mix of vivid moments and just...fog), and gave her my prepared speech.

"A couple of weeks ago I found a lump in my left breast. The biopsy results came back today and it turns out it is cancer."

Silence. Then a stuttering of "Oh my god...".

After her initial reaction we talked about the game plan, the details, the facts. She's an accountant so that was where her brain went first, and I was great with that because the facts didn't make me cry.

Then I called my older sister, or maybe she called me back, I don't remember. I gave her the same prepared sentences, and she had the same shocked silence as my younger sister had. I launched into the game plan, and she listened, but then asked gently, "How are *you* doing with all of this?" That stopped me in my tracks. I had no idea. And honestly, I don't remember how I answered her. I'm pretty sure I dissolved into a stupid sobbing mess.

I made a few more phone calls that week. Each person I talked to had a different response and asked different questions, but every single one had a stunned silence after my rehearsed sentences, so my advice to you is that you be ready for that. Their brains are doing the same thing yours did when you found out – it's on overload – and they will have no idea what to say. I wound up putting together a couple of follow-up sentences to help them focus on what I wanted them to focus on. "I don't know the plan yet, but it's in motion and they're going to attack this with everything they've got", or "I'm scared but I'm going to get through this", that kind of thing.

My third tier consisted of people who needed to find out before the Facebook crowd but didn't need a personal phone call. There are probably some folks who should have been in the second tier that got an email instead, but at some point you're just done with the phone calls. So I drafted a witty and informative email to send to good friends and my extended family – aunts, uncles, cousins, etc. I'll share it with you here.

Scary News

I'm sorry to do this via email, but I'm going to be selfish and do this in a way where I can sound incredibly steady and in control :-)

I found out Tuesday that I have breast cancer.

I'm not going to lie, it's a scary cancer - the tumor grew incredibly fast and is pretty large, and getting breast cancer before you're 40 is not something to take lightly. But I'm a stubborn bitch and a control freak, so you can be certain I'm not going anywhere, and I'm sure as hell not letting someone else raise my kids. Hell ass no. I AM going to have to go through chemotherapy & surgery, and I'm going to be pretty sick for a while - those of you who have been through cancer in one way or another know that better than I do. And I'm going to need help and support and laughter and patience and probably a wig somewhere along the way and definitely someone to come take my kids out to run around on days I can't do it myself.

For now, please keep this news between the people on this email and/or your spouses and significant others - no Facebook messages or anything public yet please. When I'm ready for that I'll post it myself and you'll know it's open to everyone. As far as the kids are concerned, they have been hearing for a couple of weeks now about how "Mommy's boobie is sick", and that's what they'll continue to hear. They have heard about some of the tests, have seen the crazy bruising and bandages from the 2 biopsies I had, but I don't plan to tell them that Mommy is sick, only that Mommy's boobie is sick. It's a little less scary that way.

I will survive this - I'm scared as hell of the chemo, and sad about losing my breast and my hair and my summer but I promise you I'm not going anywhere. And while I will support and condone and probably even join you in feeling scared and dramatic about the whole thing, I need you to keep focused on my survival. The collective thought needs to be that I will beat this. Let yourself feel whatever you need to feel, but do not spend time imagining me gone or worrying about what would happen to my kids - that only encourages the Universe to fulfill that image and I cannot allow that. And because I'm the one who's sick, I get to be weird and metaphysical and controlling of your thoughts. Actually, because I'm a mom I get to do that. My kids deserve that.

I will try and keep people posted as this whole thing progresses. I may or may not create a blog or some such nonsense to do that - not sure how to handle all of it yet. I'm on a very steep learning curve and it's a bit daunting at the moment. I will be open to any and all questions, but I'm a little overwhelmed this week, and will be for another couple of weeks as I get through all of the consultations and scans and tests and whatnot, but once things level off I'll be pretty open about everything, as I tend to be :-) Oh and in case you don't already know this about me, I'm not much of a phone person...I'm good with texts & emails & private messages on Facebook though!

Much love,

K

PS For those of you needing stats and technical terms, here you go. The cancer is still being staged - I will have a PET scan this week to determine whether it has metastasized, but I'm at a minimum of stage 2 because of the size of the tumor - the little bastard is 7cm X 5cm. Until they know whether it has metastasized, it's being considered a locally advanced breast cancer, I've also heard it referred to as invasive ductal carcinoma. I will be having a full mastectomy, possibly a double mastectomy but that part is my choice. They may or may not be able to salvage the nipple on my healthy breast, but I'm definitely losing the nipple on my left one - this is a point of sadness for me that I can't really explain, but also a good excuse for a new tattoo :-) They're going to start with surgery, probably in a couple of weeks, then look at chemo. I have a list of people I'm supposed to consult with right away - a new surgeon up in Portland (the surgeon who diagnosed me is in Salem), an oncologist, a genetic counselor and a regular mental health cancer counselor type person. That's everything I know at this point.

I am very long winded and very open about my life. You may not be the kind of person who goes into that kind of detail and obviously that's fine. But what worked about that email is that it covered everything. It gave them 1) the main information, 2) how I wanted them to support me, 3) how I wanted them to contact me, and 4) my preferences on how much they talked about it publicly. The emails I got in response weren't filled with questions I couldn't/didn't want to answer, they were just words of support and love. And that's what I needed right then. I had to teach my community how to care for me, and the best way to do that was to tell them what I needed as best I could. You may be able to do it in a much shorter email, but covering those main points will help everyone who loves you know how to respond.

Are there going to be times you have no idea what you need? Of course…oh my god of course. In those cases, just say that. "I don't know what I need." It was a steep learning curve for me, but being absolutely honest in each moment instead of trying to come up with what I thought others needed to hear (or not hear) was often the difference between a good day and a bad day.

Roughly a week after I sent the email I had made it through the PET scan, talked to Kaiser's Breast Care Navigator (think wedding planner for breast cancer – she was amazing), given the genetic counselor my family history and given blood for the BRCA gene test, and gotten the results of the second biopsy (which did not, to my chagrin, tell me that the first biopsy had been misdiagnosed and I didn't in fact have cancer). I was ready to tell the Facebook crowd. By this point some of the shock was clearing up, and with the help of my best friends and sisters I was reclaiming my humor. So I posted this:

"Little Bastard, meet Facebook friends, Facebook friends, meet Little Bastard. Little Bastard is the lump in my left breast that the doctor says is cancer. Little Bastard is a lonely little bastard, because I've caught him before he had a chance to make any bastard minions anywhere else in my body. And don't you worry Facebook friends, Little Bastard is going down hard."

I got forty-nine responses to that, all shouts and cheers of "Hell yes!", "Kill the bastard!" and "Kick its ass!" You could practically hear the crowd yelling like they were in an ultimate fighting ring.

It's good that I'm typing this and not telling the story out loud, because when I read those responses, I shake and blubber like a beauty pageant winner.

I could feel myself being lifted up and carried by their strength. That was the day my Facebook crowd became my Facebook Army. And my Facebook Army is my great weapon – we have tackled much together, and proven that the power of group prayer, even when the prayers are said within the constructs of multiple religions, is the most powerful force out there. I've got Christians,

Pagans, Mormons, Buddhists, Muslims…even the agnostics and atheists put their energies into the universe and make the earth move.

Your Kids

There are at least a gazillion books written on how to talk to your kids about cancer, and I have neither the training nor the desire to delve into child psychology here. I simply want to share with you how I handled it, and give you some ideas on where to start.

When I was diagnosed, my kids were seven and three years old. They were all I could think about – they were my first thought the moment I found the lump. They were my strength when I was scared and my weakness when I didn't want to cry. I was lucky because they were too young to understand the gravity of the word cancer, and I was unlucky because they were too young to understand why I couldn't take them to the park or take them to their friend's birthday parties during treatment.

Our little family had already been through so much – financial crisis, divorce, multiple moves. I was about to go through a year of treatments that would leave me occasionally unable to care for them, and I had no way of guaranteeing who would be the one filling in. I had no way of giving them a routine, or confidence in what was coming next. How do you prepare small children for something of that magnitude?

What I did, for better or worse, was keep them in the loop. The biopsies left my breast battered and bruised and covered in bandages, and I didn't hide that from them. We lived in a small apartment so it would have been difficult anyway. When they asked about the bruises and the bandages I told them I had a sick boobie, and that the doctor had to take some of the tissue from inside to see what kind of sickness it was. I let them feel the lump, and pointed out how hard the inside of my left breast was in comparison to my right breast. I told them that the lump is what made my boobie sick.

During the times when I couldn't hold back the tears in front of them, I would answer their questions by telling them that I was scared for my sick boobie, the same way they were scared of getting shots, but that their hugs made me feel better.

After I was diagnosed it took a while to open up to them and actually use the word cancer. But there was just a point when it was too obvious that something was up, and it was time to let them in on what was ahead. Once I knew that I was eligible to get tissue expanders placed at the same time as my mastectomy, I sat my kids down and told them that the doctors had figured out a way to fix my sick boobie – they were going to give me *new* boobies. I talked as simply as I could about how they would make owies on both boobies and take away the sick parts, then put in new boobies.

On another day I showed them a brochure on chemo hats, and explained as best I could about the medicine they were going to give me, about how it would make me very sick and very tired, and that their grandma and their daddy and sometimes other friends would be helping to take care of them. I also mentioned that it would make my hair fall out. Both of them fell into fits of laughter at that point – the thought of me without hair was hilarious to them. The brochure also had prosthetic breasts and bras, so we talked about how the tissue expanders would be small at first so I might need to use fake boobies for a while – my son thought they looked like bean bags and called them 'bean bag boobies' and that was pretty funny too.

Then I had to do it, I had to use the word. I asked my son, who is oldest, if he knew what cancer was. He said no, but once I described it a bit he started to cry, and said he was afraid I would die.

No one can prepare you for that feeling; that helplessness and fear and strength and resolve all rolled into one.

I told him that my death was not in the plan. I told him I was going to fight as hard as I could and stick around as long as I could. I told him, "I'm going to kick cancer in the butt. Then I'm going to throw one of my bean bag boobies at it." I was careful not to make any promises about my survival, and we found things to laugh at.

Later that week we met with a family counselor in Kaiser's oncology department – the kids' daddy joined us so everyone would be on the same page. She gave us lots of reading material and talked with our son a little, but he doesn't really open up to strangers much. She gave us things to think about and some ideas on how to approach everything, and for our family that one visit was plenty. I know other families who were able to find a counselor who made a great and wonderful difference in their kids' lives, and it's something we may still look into for the future. During treatment however, we took her advice and left it at that.

Once everything went into full swing we just took each day as it came. They went to their Papa & Grammy's house in Reno for two weeks when I had my mastectomy. When they came back they learned how to give gentle hugs and how to snuggle next to me without hurting me. They loved to fetch things for me and do adult things like make their own sandwiches and pour their own milk.

You can't anticipate everything though, and there were surprises. I thought I had covered everything where my mastectomy was concerned, but when the kids wanted to see my new boobies and I showed them, my daughter started to cry. I thought maybe the wounds were too graphic for her, but what had upset her was that I didn't have nipples. It had never occurred to me to prepare her for that, but boobies without nipples scared her more than anything.

Before I started chemo we talked about germs and washing hands and keeping the toilet lid down when we flush. During chemo there were fights about having friends over, struggles over homework, and tears (from everyone) on the nights I couldn't put them to bed because I wasn't able to get out of mine. We had moved in with my mother by that point, so they had lots of time with her and she was able to pick up the slack, thank goodness. On some days they forced me to get up and deal with life when I really didn't want to, on others they climbed into bed with me and snuggled the pain and fear away.

We watched a *lot* of My Little Pony.

If you've got kids, find literature on age appropriate ways of talking with them, see if your insurance covers family counseling, and talk to teachers and caregivers about your situation. Be honest with them, and honest with yourself about what you can handle.

If your kids are little, you will need help. Be sure to set up a list of people you can call for that help – even if you have a spouse living with you (that person can't do it all, much as they might try). When friends ask if there's anything they can do, include "take my kids out to play" in your answer. It's difficult to admit it, difficult to ask for it, but this is part of your journey, part of what the Universe thinks you need to learn. Ask for what you need, ask for what your kids need, and keep asking until someone says yes.

Kindred Spirits

"Friendship isn't about who you've known the longest. It's about who came, and never left your side."

Going through cancer treatment can leave you feeling very alone. Whether you're surrounded by family and friends or not, there are things you're going through that most of them can't possibly understand. Sometimes I would listen to my friends or coworkers talking about their problems and just shake my head – they had every right to their complaints but it was just nothing in comparison to what was on my plate. Or I would try and join in a conversation and something would pop out of my mouth about PET scans or the constant blood draws and it would stop the whole conversation.

The only thing worse than listening to problems less life-threatening than yours, is the look of pity and fear that appears on everyone's face as soon as it's unveiled that their problems are less life-threatening than yours.

What you need are kindred spirits – people who are going through or have gone through similar treatments and experiences. People you can complain to about surgery scars and steroid highs who will join in, not check out.

Survivors are going to come out of the woodwork when they see or hear you're fighting cancer. The woman at the grocery store checkout, the MRI technician, the person sitting next to you on the bus who notices your port. We will smile a little too hard as we pass you on the street, we'll try our best to share funny stories and not scary stories, and we'll nod in agreement and laugh as you talk about that lab tech who flinched when he saw how shot your veins are after chemo. It's like a club we're all a part of that no one wanted to join. And we all have a lifetime membership.

In the first couple of weeks after I was diagnosed, I didn't want anything to do with other survivors. I don't know that I had a clear thought about why, only that when friends would want to connect me to another friend who was a survivor I politely declined. Or thanked them but never reached out. Something about the idea of talking to other survivors deterred me.

But soon, as the shock wore off a bit and my new normal settled in, these people became a lifeline. I joined a forum on Breastcancer.org that matched those of us going through similar treatment schedules, and there were many days that those were the only people I wanted to talk to. Because here's the thing, those people are never going to hit you with an awkward silence, or look at you like you just grew another head, or think of you as "the one who has cancer". They understand things that no one else understands, and bringing up subjects like The Red Devil, or radiation burns, or those wipes they give you to disinfect yourself the night before surgery, doesn't stop the conversation. You

65

can talk about how bad the constipation is, and laugh about "chemobrain", and burst into tears over nothing at all, and they're right there with you. They've been there, or they're right there too.

One of my favorite survivor moments occurred in the reception area of my daughter's ballet school. There were four students in her class and three mothers, including myself, who sat in the comfy chairs and couches while the girls learned first position and danced to the song "Let It Go" while singing along enthusiastically. It was summer so I wore spaghetti strap tank tops most of the time, which let my port scar show. The other two mothers, Tricia and April, and I struck up easy conversation – it was a fun group. At one point Tricia pointed at my scar and asked hesitantly if I had fought cancer. When I nodded, she immediately pulled back the top of her own blouse and showed me her matching port scar. We then launched into questions about which cancer it was and nodded enthusiastically when both of us said, "Breast cancer". April was also interested in what we'd been through and joined in the conversation about tissue expanders and recovery times after our mastectomies and whatnot. It turned out Tricia and I were both due for exchange surgery (where they take out the tissue expanders and put in the permanent implants) in the next month, so we promised to keep each other posted.

A few weeks later she came to ballet class and announced that she'd had the surgery the Friday before. April and I both congratulated her and asked how it went. I asked her if they were soft and squishy like I'd hoped (I called my tissue expanders "rock boobs", because they were hard as rocks and sutured to my ribs so they didn't move). She said yes and stuck out her chest so I could feel them – which I did immediately. April asked about mine so I leaned over to her so she could feel the rock boobs, then April felt Tricia's new boobs in comparison. We were very enthusiastic as we squealed and clapped and felt each other up. I can't even imagine what the ballet school receptionist must have been thinking.

When you're ready, find those kindred spirits. Check out the online forums on cancer websites and join one that has people you feel like are "your people". Look for support groups if you prefer to talk to people in person. And when someone opens themselves up to you and tells you they're a survivor too, don't be afraid to ask for their email address or phone number. Most survivors aren't going to want to be too pushy about it, but we're around and happy to listen, offer advice, or just have a conversation that doesn't get awkward when you start in on how chemo makes everything taste like pond water.

Telling People What You Need

This is the hard part, the real work. This is the part of the journey where you learn to be honest with yourself, honest with the people close to you, then honest with yourself again. I believe this particular chunk of lessons is the reason I got cancer in the first place.

I never thought of myself as a people-pleaser, but as I went through the process of my divorce I realized I did have a tendency to smooth everything over for everyone. I minimized my problems or ignored them completely to avoid upsetting people or putting a hardship on them. As my husband and I worked through the mediation process, I watched myself give in when I shouldn't, or just borrow money to avoid having to beg for a child support payment, or lie to avoid telling him what I needed. It made my friends and family nuts.

One day I sat down and made a series of vision boards – a collection of words and pictures cut out from magazines that represented what I wanted to do or have in the next year. Things like financial freedom, strength to declare what I need and fight for it, confidence, and another shot at love. I put them into frames and hung them on the wall in my room so I'd see them every day.

Months later I was standing in front of those vision boards after having been diagnosed with stage 3 breast cancer, and I got angry. All of those things that I had hoped for, strived for, visualized and asked the universe for, and what did I get? Goddamned freaking cancer. I raged and cried and decided to take the vision boards down entirely. My plan was to throw them off of my balcony actually, but when I walked closer to them to do just that, one phrase jumped out at me.

"Be the game changer."

My intention when I put that phrase up there was to be a game changer at my job – to climb the corporate ladder to a management position so that I could support my kids and have a nice house and relax about money. The whole cancer thing had been beyond frustrating because it would delay my ability to advance out of the department I was in until after treatment.

But this time when I read those words, I saw another option. I saw an opportunity that going through this experience might give me. I saw myself being the game changer in my whole life – the game changer in my choices, my friendships, and my community. Perhaps this experience would even give me the opportunity to be a game changer in someone else's life.

More phrases on my vision boards then caught my eye; "Make more than money." "Build deeper connections." "A new chapter."

I had already learned that I wouldn't be able to shield my loved ones from my diagnosis. I couldn't make it so that their daughter, sister, or best friend didn't have cancer. I couldn't spin it to make it look like it wasn't a big deal. And I knew I would have to learn to ask for what I needed without backing down, since a lot of what I was going to need wasn't going to be optional.

Now, looking at my vision boards, suddenly I realized that cancer was going to put me on the road to receiving everything I asked for. It was going to teach me to be honest, open, and unwavering in my convictions. I realized that cancer was, in a twisted monkey's paw kind of way, the answer to my prayers.

What cancer was going to give me was a big fat reason to think of myself first.

Divide and Conquer

So how did I break into telling people what I need? Slowly, and with a lot of internal arguments. I had to force myself to hit "send" when I was texting someone asking for their help, or even just accepting an offer of help. I had to stop myself mid-sentence and start over, this time being honest about how I was feeling. I said things like, "Tell me if this is too much…" a lot, then stopped myself and just said, "Thank you."

Most people will be more comfortable if they know you're going to be straightforward and ask for what you need. I know that's true for me – if someone I love clearly needs something but won't ask for it and won't accept my help it makes me crazy. Don't make people drag the truth out of you, it only adds to their load.

Start with the easy stuff – join a cancer forum or cancer support group and vent to them about things you're too scared to vent to friends and family about. Be honest about what you're feeling, no matter how crazy it sounds. You'll find in those places that other survivors will sigh with relief and thank you for saying it out loud, because they've been feeling the same way.

Each group of people and each person in your life has the ability to help you in a different way. Try and recognize what each person brings to the table, and go to them for those things. Your spouse cannot fulfill every need you have; neither can your mother, or your best friend or your kids. Each person close to you has something they're particularly good at, and things they will drop the ball on.

I have a wonderful group of friends that I've known since college, and every single one of them has their strengths and weaknesses. My family is very close too, and each member is someone I can go to for different things.

Having my friend Heather around is like having a mama bear in the house. If someone is bothering you she will take them out, no questions asked. She's also brutally and bluntly honest with the people she loves. She is the one who told me to get over myself when I was worried about how my diagnosis would affect other people. She's also the one I brought with me to my last surgery so she could do battle with the recovery nurse if necessary.

My cousin Kenneth had been through cancer treatment of his own, so he had first-hand knowledge of how much it sucks. He would send little messages of encouragement and bits of advice along the way. He's the one who first told me, "You've got this."

My friend Molly was like my little shiny beacon of light. She would email me virtual flowers and send funny quotes and snarky comments about boobs. She could make me laugh when no one else could. Toward the end of my treatment her son was diagnosed with Hodgkin's Lymphoma, and suddenly we had some awful things in common.

She's still my beacon of light and my favorite source for snarky boob references, but she's also the person I can talk to about cancer without having to think about whether I've talked about cancer too much lately.

My friend Chris is my spiritual touchstone. She and I share a lot of the same beliefs, and when I was ready to tackle the spiritual side of my journey, she was the one I called. She and I also have a history of saying the wrong things to each other – when her late husband was sick I would call and do my best to lift her up and help her stay positive, but I could always tell that it just wasn't right. And during my divorce the same thing would happen the other direction. What we learned is that we don't always say the right thing, but what we can do is be there for each other. She went to every chemo treatment with me; sometimes we'd talk the whole time, sometimes we'd just crochet or play solitaire on our phones. But her presence kept me grounded.

My older sister Kim was my rock and my teddy bear – something about having my big sister close made me feel safe. I could cry with her, and not worry about looking like I was weak or like I had given up. And she would turn around and call me a glowworm during the PET scan, or laugh about my T-rex arms after my mastectomy, and for just a few minutes at least, cancer was hilarious instead of terrifying.

My younger sister Kathy is the funniest, most direct person I know. I never have to worry about whether I'll get the truth from her. She was another little beacon of light for me, because no matter what, she would have a funny story or crazy opinion to share and make us all laugh.

My mom…how do I even go into how much my mom did for me? She took me and my kids in, cooked for us, helped with laundry and vacuuming when I was broken or sick, played Who Can Scare Who First with my kids, and listened to all of my rambling thoughts every day. No one has lived through the experience with me quite as much as she has.

My friends Kelly and Carrie were my escape. We have a standing dinner and play date with all of our kids every Friday, and every week during treatment, no matter how sick I was, I went. We talked a bit about what I was going through, but mostly we talked about everything else. We talked about their jobs, and laughed at our kids, and compared crushes on Sam and Dean from the show Supernatural. For one night a week, I wasn't The Friend Who Has Cancer, I was just me.

There were many others, some of whom said exactly what I needed to hear at that moment, some of whom said things that left me feeling like maybe I should try someone else for that particular subject. Each person had something to give, either in the form of helpful advice or a lesson learned about opening up to that particular person about that particular subject.

It's okay to divide and conquer when it comes to your friends and family. If nothing else, you lesson the burden on everyone by spreading out who you go to for what. But it also gives you the best chance for success – go to each person in your community for something that they're good at. And if you go to them and don't get the response you were hoping for, be honest. Tell them what response you were looking for and give them the chance to change their tactics – don't forget, they're on a learning curve too.

And if you leave the encounter feeling unresolved and frustrated, try again later, or try again with someone else.

If you don't ask, the answer is always no.

Accepting Help

You know that feeling when someone offers their help and you think, "That would be nice, but it would be such a hardship for them..." This is the time when you have to suck it up and say, "Yes, actually that would be really helpful, thank you."

Letting people help you is incredibly important. You absolutely cannot do this by yourself. If you're like me, and you're in the beginning of all this, you are probably thinking, "Screw you, yes I can." But I promise you cannot. At the very least there will be certain scans and treatments you won't be allowed to drive yourself to and from, at the most you might have small children like I did, and will need help caring for them during the tough weeks. In the middle is a hand to hold during appointments, someone to do the vacuuming every so often, and a sympathetic ear when the hats are too hot and the scarves are too bulky and the wigs just itch.

You're going to have to learn to say, "Yes, thank you."

If you're the caretaker type, or the do-it-all-yourself type and the above paragraphs have just sent your blood pressure skyrocketing, then think of it this way – letting people help you will help them.

Toward the end of my chemotherapy, the eight-year-old son of two of my best friends was diagnosed with Hodgkin's Lymphoma. Getting this news was devastating to all of us, but knowing with vivid detail what he was about to endure put me into an emotional spiral. I had harbored a somewhat vain notion that what I had been going through would keep those I love from ever having to go through it too. I was carrying that flag so that no one else would have to.

Now a kid barely old enough to have a crush on a girl was about to face the scans, the endless blood draws, the nausea and fatigue...he was about to face *cancer*. And his parents, oh my god his parents. I have never wanted to take something away from two people more in my entire life.

But I couldn't. I couldn't turn back time and give them a different diagnosis, I couldn't take away that phone call. And as much as I tried, I couldn't paint chemo a lighter color. And his mom knew it, she'd been one of my closest companions during my treatment. She knew exactly what her son was about to go through.

It was the only time I really regretted how open and honest I'd been about everything.

What made me feel better was helping. I made "warrior bracelets" for him to wear to the scans to help him feel stronger. I showed up and gave hugs in the waiting room any time I could, and I drove down and shaved his head for him when his hair started to fall out – we have a "twinsies" picture of the two of us without hair. They even let me put together a fund-raising campaign to help with medical bills. I couldn't take anything away, but I could do those things and that kept me sane. Each time I was able to contribute in some way I felt better – less helpless.

The people who love you are feeling that helplessness right now, and many will gratefully do things like come clean your kitchen or bring you food. Some folks may be willing and able to go with you to appointments and treatments. Some may have the ability to help out with your kids.

The important thing is to recognize that it's not selfish to ask for help in your current situation, it's actually somewhat generous. Even folks who can't physically be there for you can listen on a bad day or offer a word of encouragement or advice. It's imperative that you allow that, and be careful not to assume the people around you (no matter how many accidentally ignorant things are coming out of their mouths) aren't wanting to contribute in some way. The trick is letting them know what would be helpful.

Everyone needs their bathroom cleaned and a stocked freezer, I don't care who you are.

Obviously I am not suggesting that you make a list of everything you need taken care of and hand it out to the people around you expecting them to drop everything and be at your beck and call. Of course not. There are going to be people close to you who can't handle what you're going through, and people close to you who drop the ball or don't realize the severity of your situation. There are also just selfish, clueless people out there. But the ones who offer help, the ones who don't seem to know what to say but clearly care about you very much…it's okay to lean on them.

It's okay to just say, "Yes, thank you."

By the end of my treatment I felt overwhelmed about how much everyone had contributed. I couldn't believe how much my community had come together and carried me through that year. What blew my mind though, is how often I'd hear them thanking me. Thanking me for my honesty, my candor, for sharing my experience with them (I posted on Facebook a *lot*). Thanking me for being a survivor, for not letting cancer break me.

By accepting their help, I allowed them in, allowed them to learn through my experiences. Allowed them to contribute to my healing and therefore give them something to *do*. Letting them help me helped them. And also happened to keep me sane when my carpet started growing things, but I wasn't healed enough from surgery to push a vacuum.

Appointments

I was incredibly fortunate when I was diagnosed – I had a plethora of friends and family around, all of whom were singularly focused on giving me whatever I needed. I was able to pick and choose who came with me to all of the different appointments, and never felt obligated to have someone there for fear they'd be insulted. If you have that opportunity I highly suggest you make use of it – different people have different energies, and different treatments will give you different emotional reactions.

My feelings about chemo were entirely different than my feelings about surgery, for example. I was grateful that my older sister could come with me to the chemo consultation, because the mere mention of chemo left me shaking and whimpering – so having my big sister next to me made me feel safe. But when it came time for the surgery consult, I really wanted my friend Molly with me, because she's funny and crass and would be able to match wits with the cocky surgeon who had an ego the size of Texas.

My mom went with me to see the genealogist because she knew most of the family history. My friend Chris went with me to every chemo treatment, which still blows my mind. She kept me entertained, let me cry and didn't take offense when I was so sick by the time we got into her car to leave that I couldn't focus on a word she was saying.

I know survivors who didn't have a choice about who went with them to appointments and treatments, or who had to go alone. Sometimes that turns out to be a good thing – I've found that the Universe tends to put us into situations which we need, whether we think so at the time or not. But if given a choice, think carefully about who you bring with you – having someone you trust in the room can make a world of difference. Whether it's someone who takes really good notes (you'll be surprised how much you think you'll remember that utterly disappears the moment you get out of the exam room), or someone who will be able to keep you laughing, or someone who will stay strong when what the doctors are saying gets the better of you.

Sometimes I brought someone specifically because they had experience in whatever specialty I was going to – my sister had been through plastic surgery before, for example, so I was grateful to have her with me for the reconstruction consult because she asked questions I wouldn't have thought of. Or during chemo treatments, Chris could translate certain things for me because she had been through chemo with her late husband. She would also write down the questions I rambled on about during treatments, then bring them up to my oncologist at the next check-up.

Something that came out of bringing a bunch of different people with me to my initial

81

appointments (that I didn't even think about until I was looking back on it), is that I was bringing my friends and family with me on my journey too. They weren't just coming along to keep me company, they were living through all of this *with* me. My closest friends and family were there in the trenches by my side, not just hearing stories about it.

I didn't bring someone with me to everything – I did radiation almost entirely by myself, and that's how I wanted it. For whatever reason, that part of treatment was just something I needed to face alone. I was grateful to have a choice in the matter and do what felt right at the time.

Don't underestimate the importance of recognizing how you feel about each piece of this journey, and who you want to take with you for the different components. You'll be surprised at how much of a difference the right person sitting beside you can make.

"You Did NOT Just Say That..."

When Strangers Say Stupid Things

People are stupid. As a rule, we are ignorant, clumsy, easily panicked animals who jump to conclusions and blurt out inappropriate things all the time. That said, we are also capable of great compassion, generosity, and selflessness. There are people out there who swerve to purposefully hit an animal with their car, and people who will cross a busy highway on foot to try and save a dog trapped on the median. There are just no limits to what we as a species are capable of.

Talk to any cancer survivor and they'll have their stories. The things people said to them that left them dumbfounded and hurt. The people they thought were close who withdrew in fear of saying the wrong thing. The things perfect strangers felt were appropriate to tell them in the middle of the grocery store. We've all got the stories, so will you. You probably have a couple already.

In those moments right after the incredibly dumb thing has been said, you have a few choices. You can react, and say exactly how dumb that person is and how hurtful what they said was.

83

That's not *always* the wrong way to go – I found that when my stress levels were high and it was a stranger in a public place, taking that option let off a little steam and helped me feel better for a few minutes at least. Of course then guilt would inevitably needle its way in, so the good feelings didn't usually last.

Another option is to smile and say thank you ("Yes, of course I wanted to hear about your friend who died last year of the same cancer I have, how did you know?"), but unless you are much more enlightened than I am, that option will eat at you and you'll yell at them in your head for days afterward.

The route I found to be best was absolute honesty. To the point, open honesty with as much of a gentle edge as I could muster. Let them know that what they just said hurt and why, but if possible without accusations or name calling. A teachable moment, so to speak.

A couple of examples:

"I know you want to share, but what I need to focus on right now is my survival and recovery."

"I'm so sorry to hear about your friend. My story is not the same as hers/his, and I'm working pretty hard to focus on survival instead of death right now."

In addition to the outbursts of random things you'll also have to deal with awkward silences. If you're in the middle of chemo and have no hair and a sallow complexion you probably won't have to "out" yourself as a cancer patient, because it will be obvious just looking at you. But if you haven't lost your hair yet, or you wear a wig, or if you're on a treatment that lets you keep your hair, then there may be moments when you have to decide if you're going to tell the people you're standing in front of that you are fighting cancer. And if you decide to go ahead and tell them, then you'll inevitably have a few awkward silences. The people who go silent are most likely not judging you, it's doubtful that they're disgusted by you or scared of you – if they're able to think anything clearly at all they're probably terrified of saying the wrong thing. Their minds are either blank or screaming, "What do I say what do I say what do I say?!?!!"

You'll have to be patient with this. It's also a good idea to take an internal temperature before you out yourself and make sure you're feeling like you can handle an awkward silence if that's what happens.

I can't tell you how to fill that silence, because it all depends on why you wanted to tell that person you're fighting cancer in the first place. Sometimes I just say, "Anyway..." and keep talking about the subject that brought up my cancer story. Sometimes I let them have a moment and just say, "It's okay." I've found a few go-to sentences that feel rehearsed because I've said them so much, but they seem to work to get us past the awkward moment. "It's just a crappy year, then I'll be done." "I've learned so much through this experience that I wouldn't trade it for anything." "I'm just grateful it's me going through this and not my kids." Sometimes though, when it was a crappy day or week, I just blurted out the truth, "Yeah, it sucks and I really hate this part of treatment. So what I was saying…"

As you go through the process of telling people about your diagnosis you'll start to find what works for you. My "theme" all the way through treatment is that I wasn't going to waste the experience – I was going to come out of this as strong as I've ever been. And a huge part of that was being honest with people. I've always been the kind of person who smoothed things over for the people in my life, kept the ugly parts hidden under a smile and a joke and a "Don't worry, I'll take care of it".

But cancer didn't let me do that. I couldn't make it go away, I couldn't get through it alone, and I couldn't make it sound less scary by describing it differently. So I have had to learn how to be honest, how to be open, and how to ask for what I need. That means taking a good look inside each time I'm presented with the option of telling someone I fought cancer. If I'm feeling a little vulnerable that day, I hold my tongue.

Because people are stupid.

"Okay...Good Talk..."

When People Close to You Say Stupid Things

The people in your life want to help. They want to make you feel better, or at the very least lesson your load. The people who love you want to make your diagnosis and treatment go away, they want to reverse time and change events so that you are no longer going through this. The people who love you might even wish they could do all of this for you. These people sit in their cars and cry for you, they think of you when they wake up in the morning and wish over and over that you weren't going through this. I've been on both sides of the experience, and I can tell you with certainty that at least one person in your life finds themselves in tears when they think of your diagnosis and treatment.

Because of this, because of their intense love for you, you are going to have to forgive them sometimes. If this is their first experience with cancer, their first experience with someone close to them going through a major illness, you are going to have to forgive them a lot. Because people are stupid and don't know what to say, because people are stupid and don't realize what not to say. And because every person is different, there are going to be things said that you couldn't have possibly predicted would hurt you. So you'll have to learn to be honest with yourself, and then honest with the people around you. And then you'll have to forgive.

Part of having a community is accepting people for who they are. You can't change a person, not really, and if someone is self-absorbed or unaware, you won't be able to change that. But you *can* gently point out the things that are hurtful, and in doing so help yourself. By practicing the art of being honest with your feelings and then honest with the people around you, you have the opportunity to grow in a way that will change your life forever.

One thing I noticed right after I let people know about my diagnosis is that everyone started walking on eggshells around me. I could tell that they had a million questions, a million worries, and that they wanted to be able to joke about things (something my community thrives on) but didn't know what was appropriate. We all, as a group, had to figure it out. And the only way we could do that was for me to remain 100% honest. If something someone said was over the top or hurt me in some way, I told them. Then that person and I could talk about it and figure out a new boundary.

When it comes to jokes, everyone has different limits. The biggest thing you need to do is set the precedent. If you joke about cancer, then the people around you will feel free to joke as well. If you think cancer jokes are abysmal and inappropriate, then most people will pick up on that and refrain. Your community is like an audience right after the house lights dim – they're waiting for you to set the stage and tell them how to react. So do that – say what you're thinking, what you're feeling, and stay honest.

Some of the jokes my friends made were really funny. Some were out of control and not funny at all. For the latter, I tried to respond with a simple "Ouch" so that we all knew a line had been crossed, but still felt safe joking around. I found that the more honest I was about what was funny and what wasn't, the safer my friends felt about making jokes and keeping moments light – they knew if they crossed a line that I'd tell them.

The other issue I ran into were the people who had such a large reaction to my diagnosis that I found myself comforting them instead of the other way around. If you find yourself saying things to your friends and family like, "It's going to be okay" or "It's not a big deal", stop right there. It's not your job to comfort them, or to make things less of a big deal so that they aren't as affected. It's not possible to do that anyway – you cannot make it so that their friend/family member doesn't have cancer. They are going to feel pain, and will need to be comforted, but not by you. If you're the caretaking type and can't just back away, then maybe suggest other people close to you whom they can talk to. Or enlist another friend or family member who can check in with that person and take the load off of you. Don't get swept up in their reaction - you've got enough to think about and feel on your own. In this instance it's perfectly okay to say, "I love you, and I want you to have the support you need, it just can't be me holding you up right now." Or even excuse yourself from the conversation entirely.

A fellow cancer survivor told me how his sister was so upset about his diagnosis that she started wailing and even dropped to her knees in anguish right in front of him. Another survivor told the story of how her ex-husband would burst into tears every time he came over to pick up their kids for the weekend. You'll probably end up with at least one person who you seem to be comforting as though they're the one going through cancer treatment, and of course how you handle it will depend on your relationship with them. I suggest being honest with them if possible, and avoiding them if not.

There are also those times when it's nice to get out of your own pity party for a while, and self-absorbed friends can be perfect for those situations. Engage them in a conversation about their life and take a break from your own.

The more you treat uncomfortable moments as "teachable moments", the better things will get as time goes on. I don't expect you to be Mary freaking Poppins all the time, especially when you're sick and scared and don't have any idea why someone talking about their cat just sent you into a sobbing fit. Just don't hide that it happened, or stuff it down inside so that your friends don't have a chance to learn how to say the right things. If the story about your friend's cat made you cry, let them know. Figure it out together, or at the very least get to the point you can laugh together about the fact that a story about a cat caught in the couch turned you into a sobbing mess.

They love you, and they *want* to say the right things. But they're people, and as I've said, people are stupid. So be honest with yourself, then honest with them. And if you can, forgive them.

Toxic People

"The way to win with a toxic person is not to play."

Hopefully most of the people in your life are both brilliant and positive, and always say the right thing, or have good intentions but just flub it up sometimes. Hopefully everyone around you is rallying and cheering you on. That's not always the case, however. Unfortunately, it's possible to have someone in your life who doesn't have your back, who refuses to be positive. Someone who says hurtful things and then defends their right to say them. Someone who is just toxic.

If someone close to you says hurtful things on a regular basis, or refuses to get on board with how serious what you're going through is, they may be someone whom you should consider toxic. This is a person who doesn't really have your best interests at heart, someone who drags you down every time you talk to them, and who doesn't change their behavior, no matter how honest you are with them.

I've talked ad nauseum about forgiving the people close to us who say stupid things. But you cannot treat a toxic person the same as a regular person. You have to find a way to put up a barrier between you and a toxic person, or eject them from your life entirely.

If this is a distant aunt or a friend on Facebook, that can be quite easy.

But often, in the stories I've heard, the toxic person is one of those who are closest to the person going through treatment. Their husband, sister, parent etc. Someone they can't just walk away from.

If you have a toxic person in your life and can't get space between you and them on your own, I encourage you to seek counseling and talk to someone specifically about your situation. This is not the time to forgive and put up with being constantly hurt and brought down. This is a time when you need as much positivity and reinforcement as you can get. If counseling isn't an option, seek out someone you can at least vent to – maybe someone on a cancer forum or in a cancer support group.

Because despite what one toxic person told a friend of mine, this *is* all about you and what you need.

Your Medical Team

Regardless of your type of cancer and the treatments recommended for it, you will find yourself surrounded by a lot of medical folk. Each specialty brings its own positives and negatives, and learning to accept each doctor's social strengths and weaknesses is important. So is recognizing a bad fit, and switching doctors if necessary.

I found that the people in oncology are an incredible breed. From the doctors and physician's assistants to the nurses, pharmacists and phlebotomists they're just different. Perhaps it's something about the length of time patients have to deal with this disease; maybe it just draws professionals with empathy and a natural kindness. An honest kindness – no one tries to snow you or paint a picture that's prettier than the reality. They're like, "Yes, this will hurt. Take my hand and I'll be here the whole way."

When I meet with my oncologist, I never feel hurried. He listens to stories about my kids with just as much interest as stories about my chemo side effects. He explains things in a calm, precise manner, and doesn't make me feel like I'm nuts when I bring up fears or questions.

My mastectomy surgeon, on the other hand, was cocky and loud and hurried through every appointment. He was also funny, and his confidence in himself made me feel confident in what he was about to do. I had to have a list of questions written down and ready to go or I wasn't going to be able to ask them, and I couldn't vent to him about fears that he couldn't fix. I'm used to surgeons being cocky and arrogant though, and actually tend to trust them more when they are, so he was a good fit for me.

There was a cocky and arrogant oncologist that I had to see a couple of times when my oncologist was unavailable, and I complained about him to anyone and everyone who would listen – and I requested that I not have to see him again. Cocky and arrogant surgeons are a good fit for me, cocky and arrogant oncologists are not.

It's always okay to get a second opinion, and switch doctors if necessary.

Nurses should get a whole book to themselves, because they are the ones beside you at every step – my love for nurses cannot be measured. When I delivered my daughter, it was a nurse who pulled me out of my blind panicked screams. When they took my breasts, it was a nurse in the pre-op room who was honest with me about what recovery would be like, who let me cry and admit how ashamed I was that the tumor could get so big without me knowing. And every week in the chemo infusion room, it was the nurses who chatted with me and laughed with me and knew what I was going through, because they were in the trenches talking to patients every day.

I respect their space by not rummaging through the cabinets in the exam rooms (okay fine, I did once when I needed a tissue…but I apologized when I got caught). I chat with them, but try not to launch into a long story or an endless list of what sucks about that particular treatment – I know that they are usually on a bit of a time crunch, and have to stay emotionally shielded to survive their job. And I make sure I thank them profusely for all of their hard work. It's not the worst idea to have friends or family bring cookies for the nurses' station if you're staying in the hospital.

Because of the sheer volume of nurses that you're likely to come across, the law of averages says that at least once you'll be faced with one who is outright mean, or having a crappy day and willing to take it out on you. I find that quietly standing up for myself in those instances has the most success – I avoid insults but hold my ground. Nurses have a job to do and don't need you getting in their way unnecessarily, but it is your body and you are a person, not just a patient.

There are innumerable other medical professionals that you'll cross paths with, and while most will be in and out of your life in an instant, sometimes you'll have an unexpected encounter that will brighten your day and stay with you for a long time. They'll have kind words or shared stories or just say that one thing that makes a difference.

Every part of your medical team has an essential role, and should be a good fit for you. The same way you should be picky about who comes with you to appointments, it's okay to be picky about who you go see. If you meet with an oncologist that you don't trust or whom you can't imagine opening up to about your fears and your pain and, let's face it, your poop, find another one.

If you're staying in the hospital and a nurse is being really cranky, ask for someone different (or better yet, have a friend or family member do it). Treat them with respect and demand that they do the same.

And bring cookies whenever possible.

Jealousy

*"Calamities are of two kinds: misfortune to
ourselves, and good fortune to others."*
~Ambrose Bierce

I've found a new thing to be upset and
jealous of lately – women who've had
mastectomies whose scars are much smaller than
mine. My incision lines run all along the bottom of
my breast, with another line up to where my nipple
used to be. I don't really understand why they
fileted me the way they did, when other women's
scars are just a short line across the middle. I
shouldn't complain too much, it's possible that
because he used such large incisions my surgeon
was able to spot the abnormal lymph nodes (the
initial sentinel-node biopsy came back clean – if he
hadn't noticed the nodes that didn't look right, they
might have sewn me up and sent me on my way
with six undiagnosed metastasis). It's just hard to
see reconstruction pictures of women where you
can't even freaking find the scars, then look in the
mirror and see what feels like horrible deformities.

You're going to have so many things to be
jealous of – people who haven't been through
hardship (or at least don't appear to have been
through hardship), people with hair, people whose

98

cancer and treatment were less severe than yours, people with out-of-pocket maximums that are less than yours.

I'm here to tell you that's okay. Don't let it eat you up inside or anything, but it's okay. It's natural, and part of the mourning process. Your life has been turned upside down – of course you're going to be envious of people who are still floating on an even keel.

If you find that you're fixating on the things other people have or don't have to deal with, then it doesn't take much searching on the internet or news channels to find people in much worse scenarios than you. Then you can feel gratitude that their problems aren't your problems.

There's generally always someone around who is worse off than you, in one way or another.

I have three friends who all had kids around the same time I did, and we have a hierarchy when it comes to swapping birth stories. One friend was in labor a handful of hours, and pushed for about ten minutes. I was in labor longer than her, and pushed for forty-five minutes, so if she and I are together I get to complain more than her. Another friend pushed for two hours and wound up having to have a stage three episiotomy, so if she's in the room I get to shut up and be grateful. Our third friend pushed for two hours, then went in for an emergency caesarean, which then had complications because the baby was stuck in the birth canal. When she's around, *no one* gets to gripe about their birth story.

You are truly never given anything the Universe doesn't think you can handle. My hope is that when you get to the other side of this experience, you'll be able to see that.

After all, that woman with the perfectly shaped breasts might look that way because she had to have her real ones cut off. You never know.

Your New Normal

I'm not going to lie to you, I still struggle with my New Normal. I've said over and over that I don't want to waste this experience – that to truly gain everything I can from my cancer experience I have to change my life and walk this new path.

But it's scary.

I'll never be the same person I was the day before my diagnosis. My identity changed, my goals changed. And most importantly my priorities changed. I no longer shrink from my dreams, or tell people what they want to hear. I no longer make dumb excuses for why I can't or couldn't do something, because now I understand the difference between an actual obstacle and just not wanting to do something.

But to do that, to live that way, I'm forging a very new path. And it's not a path that is particularly familiar to me, or always comfortable.

I'm also acutely aware at all times of the changes in my body. There are the obvious changes like my fake boobs and my short hair and the constant hot flashes. But there are other changes that aren't as obvious – my nails aren't as strong as they used to be, and the neuropathy that showed up when I was on taxol hasn't disappeared completely, so I have one toe on my left foot I can't always feel.

Constant reminders of what I've been through.

When I finished chemotherapy and was in the "healing period" before radiation started, I was flooded with emotions. For five months I had lived in a very specific reality – I had been "on chemo". When I could no longer identify with that reality, I didn't feel like I knew who I was supposed to be. I knew I was supposed to be healing, but what did that look like? I didn't know how to heal when I was outside of a chemo cycle – I'd created a routine around getting just well enough for the next treatment. Now I wasn't 100% healed but I wasn't a mess; I wasn't "on chemo" but I wasn't completely away from the side effects yet, and I wasn't done either – I still had radiation and then reconstructive surgeries ahead. I was supposed to be celebrating but I couldn't gather an emotion even close to that.

I started really identifying with soldiers who came home and then just turned around and went back to war. I was supposed to be happy to be done, but a large part of me just wanted to go back to where it was familiar, where I knew who I was supposed to be and what I was supposed to be doing. Where the choices were clear – life or death – and there were people around me facing exactly the same thing.

After radiation ended and I was told I would have to wait at least six months to start reconstructive surgeries, I nearly panicked. Suddenly I was left out in the cold – no longer in cancer treatment, but forever changed and unable to simply go back to my old life.

My friends threw a "Cancer Free" party, my Facebook page blew up with congratulations and cheering, everyone celebrated. Everyone but me.

I can't tell you how to get through this period. What I can tell you is that it's normal, you're not crazy, and you're not alone. And it will end. At some point your motor will start back up again and you'll move forward into your future with a steady heart.

And the things you've learned along the way are going to keep serving you. You can now look something scary in the face and keep moving forward regardless of how afraid you are. And no matter the current state of your body, you are mentally stronger than you've ever been.

Maybe you're like me and after treatment all you have to worry about is recurrence. Maybe you're looking at a lifetime of intermittent treatments. Either way you're no longer the person you were. Hearing or seeing the word cancer lights up a different part of your brain than it used to. If you can bring that into your life as a positive reinforcement, then your New Normal can be really beautiful.

When it comes to your community, you're different too. Good, bad or ugly you are now The One Who Had Cancer. You're a little bit more famous than you were before. There may be higher expectations of you too – do you feel somehow obligated to do the next "cancer run" or watch and report on the show where the lead character has cancer? I do. I have to be careful to hold certain boundaries so I don't open emotional wounds.

Going to see the movie "A Fault in Our Stars" was a bad idea, for example. But starting to write about what I've been through has been very therapeutic.

Anniversaries might be hard – I was a complete mess for several of them. The anniversary of the day I found the lump, the anniversary of my diagnosis, my mastectomy, the first day of chemo. Each one was unexpectedly emotional. The thing about anniversaries is, you aren't in the middle of it anymore. You don't have to be strong and resilient and stoic anymore. You've done it, you lived through it and lived through the twelve months that followed, and now you can look back and...feel everything. The anniversaries are, in a weird way, harder than the events themselves, because the crisis is over and you can fall apart now without jeopardizing your recovery.

My best advice is to feel it, let yourself have those emotions, forgive yourself for getting lost in a memory. Let that day be significant if you need to. Then remember the lessons cancer has taught you, and put one foot in front of the other again.

Out in the world there will be stories you want to tell a new acquaintance, and you'll realize halfway through that there's no way you can tell it properly without dropping the C-bomb. Then you'll get to face the decision of whether to 'out' yourself as a cancer survivor. You'd think it would get easier each time, but it hasn't for me. Sometimes it's uncomfortable and stops the conversation, and makes me feel like I just put a giant flashing sign on my forehead that says, "Cancer Girl". Other times I find a new friend because it turns out we have something in common.

Your New Normal will change as you go; on some days you might feel sorry for yourself and jealous of the people who haven't been through what you've been through; other days you might feel nothing but gratitude for the shift in your reality which cancer brought. When I look at the way I was living my life before my diagnosis – the anger and resentment and stress I carried every day, I'm not surprised the Universe needed to pick me up and put me on another path. But I'm not perfect – I get a little annoyed at women who complain about their long hair, and I'm jealous to the point of rage at *everyone* who still has nipples.

It's a New Normal, not Enlightenment.

Allow the lessons you've learned to permeate your life. Allow yourself to be pissed off. Allow yourself to get back to your routine. Allow yourself to scrap that routine and completely forge a new path. Allow yourself time to mourn. Allow allow allow.

Your New Normal is whatever you want it to be. Truly.

Conclusion

"The difference between 'try' and 'triumph'...is a little 'umph'"

You've got this. You can do it, and you are strong enough for anything that you encounter along the way.

I hope this book has given you some tools to use as you get through your cancer journey. I won't lie to you; it's not going to be easy. There are going to be hard days, and really hard days. You are being dragged into something that not everyone is strong enough to handle.

But *you* are. You are absolutely strong enough to handle this. Just the fact that you read this book shows me you are, because you're *willing* to be. You're out there looking for inspiration and help, and that tells me you'll be just fine. Put together your SOS's and use them when you need. Laugh whenever you can, and forgive yourself when you can't.

I wish for you the very best during your cancer treatment. I give you blessings of strength, resilience, good friends, and a new look on life.

You've got this, you really do.

Acknowledgments

I am profoundly thankful to the following people for their support, advice, and inspiration during my journey: Molly & Mitch Jones, Christina Safford, Heather O'Mara, Blaise Cook-Baron, Kim & Charles Leddon, Kathy & Matt Germer, Bonnie Jones, Kelly McCord, Carrie Heiberger, Ken & Amber Freitas, Tina Allen, Cecil Averett, Cecil M. & Cathy Averett, A.J. Voytko, and Wayne Singer.

I am also incredibly grateful for everyone in my Facebook Army, and for the ladies on the Breastcancer.org forums. Without you, I would have been completely lost at sea on more than one occasion.

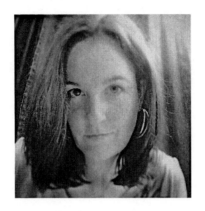

K. Susanne Jones

resides in the Pacific Northwest, where she splits her time between her two favorite things – writing, and raising her children. After surviving divorce and breast cancer, she has committed herself to helping others find inspiration via her website, www.ajonesgirl.com and her non-fiction books, which focus on self-improvement and transformation.